A
BEGINNER'S
GUIDE
TO CALISTHENICS
FOR WOMEN

Easy to Follow Workouts Suitable for
all Fitness

LIAMS BROOKS

TABLE OF CONTENTS

INTRODUCTION

The Power of Bodyweight Training

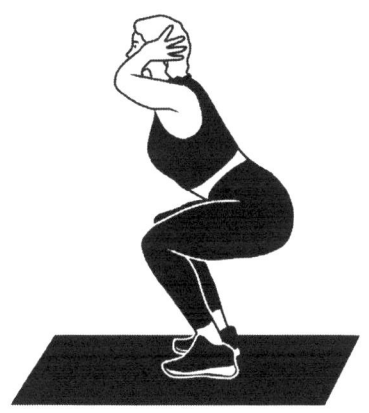

Understanding Calisthenics

Calisthenics, derived from the Greek words "kallos" meaning beauty and "sthenos" meaning strength, is a form of exercise that uses the body's weight as resistance to develop physical fitness. Unlike weightlifting, which relies on external weights, calisthenics emphasizes functional movements that can be performed anywhere, requiring minimal to no equipment. This approach to fitness is both ancient and modern, tracing its roots back to the military training regimens of ancient civilizations, where soldiers performed bodyweight exercises to build the strength, agility, and endurance needed for battle. Over centuries, calisthenics has evolved, but its core principles of using the body to master the body remain unchanged.

In recent years, calisthenics has experienced a resurgence in popularity, particularly among women, due to its accessibility and effectiveness. The rise of social media has played a significant role in this revival, with fitness enthusiasts sharing routines and showcasing impressive feats of strength and control. Calisthenics embodies a fitness philosophy that prioritizes natural movement, making it an ideal choice for those seeking to build a strong, resilient body without relying on complex gym equipment.

Benefits for Women: Strength, Flexibility, and Confidence
Calisthenics offers a range of benefits that are particularly appealing to women. One of the primary advantages is the development of functional strength.

Unlike traditional weight training, which often isolates specific muscle groups, calisthenics engages multiple muscles simultaneously, leading to improved overall strength and coordination. This is particularly beneficial for women, who may seek to build lean muscle and enhance their physical capabilities without the bulk often associated with heavy weightlifting.

Flexibility is another significant benefit of calisthenics. Many exercises, such as lunges, squats, and various yoga-inspired movements, promote both dynamic and static flexibility. This increased range of motion not only enhances performance in physical activities but also reduces the risk of injury in daily life. For women, who may face unique physical challenges such as maintaining joint health and managing the effects of aging, the flexibility gained through calisthenics can be particularly empowering.

Beyond the physical benefits, calisthenics also fosters confidence. As women progress in their calisthenics journey, they gain a greater sense of control over their bodies. Mastering challenging movements like pull-ups or handstands provides a tangible sense of accomplishment, boosting self-esteem and reinforcing the belief that they are capable of overcoming obstacles. This confidence often extends beyond the workout, influencing other areas of life and promoting a positive body image.

Debunking Myths: Common Misconceptions About Calisthenics and Women

Despite its benefits, several myths about calisthenics persist, particularly concerning its suitability for women. One common misconception is that calisthenics is too challenging for beginners or those with less upper body strength. However, calisthenics is inherently scalable, with exercises that can be modified to suit all fitness levels. For example, women new to push-ups can start with knee push-ups or wall push-ups before progressing to full push-ups.

Another myth is that calisthenics will make women overly muscular or bulky. In reality, calisthenics tends to promote lean muscle growth due to the nature of bodyweight resistance, which is less likely to lead to the hypertrophy (increase in muscle size) seen in heavy weightlifting. The emphasis on high repetitions and controlled movements in calisthenics leads to muscle endurance and toning rather than excessive muscle mass. Finally, some believe that calisthenics is less effective than traditional gym workouts. This misconception overlooks the comprehensive nature of calisthenics, which not only builds strength but also enhances balance, flexibility, and cardiovascular health. Many women find that calisthenics provides a more balanced and enjoyable approach to fitness, leading to long-term adherence and better overall health outcomes.

Getting Started

Essential Gear: Clothing and Footwear

One of the advantages of calisthenics is its minimalistic approach to equipment. However, having the right clothing and footwear can significantly enhance your comfort and performance. Opt for breathable, moisture-wicking fabrics that allow for a full range of motion. Tight-fitting clothes, such as compression leggings and fitted tops, are preferable as they reduce the risk of fabric getting caught or hindering movement during exercises.

Footwear is another crucial consideration. While some calisthenics enthusiasts prefer to train barefoot to improve balance and proprioception, others might opt for minimalistic shoes that offer a barefoot-like experience with some protection. These shoes should provide adequate grip, support, and flexibility to allow for natural foot movement. If you plan to include running or jumping exercises in your routine, choose shoes with enough cushioning to absorb impact while maintaining stability.

Setting Up a Workout Space at Home or Outdoors

Calisthenics is versatile and can be practiced almost anywhere, but having a dedicated workout space can help maintain consistency and focus. At home, a small area with enough room to stretch out fully is sufficient. You might want to invest in a yoga mat for comfort during floor exercises and a pull-up bar that can be installed in a doorway. Resistance bands and parallettes are other optional tools that can enhance your workouts as you progress.

Outdoors, parks and playgrounds offer natural environments for calisthenics. Look for spaces with flat ground, sturdy bars, and benches that can be used for a variety of exercises. Training outdoors also has the added benefits of fresh air and natural sunlight, which can boost mood and energy levels.

Goal Setting: Tracking Progress and Staying Motivated

Setting clear and realistic goals is key to staying motivated in your calisthenics journey. Start by identifying your main objectives, whether it's building strength, improving flexibility, losing weight, or simply staying active. Break these down into smaller, achievable milestones. For example, if your goal is to do a full push-up, start by aiming to complete 10 knee push-ups with perfect form.

Tracking your progress is essential to maintain motivation and measure improvement. Use a fitness journal or app to record your workouts, noting the number of sets, reps, and any modifications you made.

Regularly reviewing your progress can help you stay focused and adjust your routine as needed.

Consistency is the cornerstone of success in calisthenics. Establishing a routine that fits your lifestyle is crucial. Whether it's a quick 20-minute session in the morning or a longer workout in the evening, finding a time that works for you will help you stick to your plan. To keep things interesting, vary your exercises and challenge yourself with new movements as you become more confident.

Finally, remember that motivation can ebb and flow. Surround yourself with supportive friends or join online communities where you can share your progress, ask questions, and draw inspiration from others. Celebrate your achievements, no matter how small, and use setbacks as learning experiences to fuel your future success.

This in-depth exploration of the basics of calisthenics sets the stage for a successful and empowering fitness journey tailored specifically for women. With the right knowledge, gear, and mindset, calisthenics can be a transformative experience, enhancing not only physical strength but also mental resilience and confidence.

CHAPTER ONE

Building a Strong Foundation

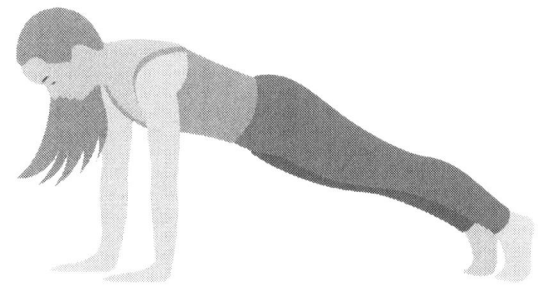

Core Principles of Calisthenics

The Importance of Proper Form and Technique

Proper form and technique are the cornerstones of effective calisthenics training. Performing exercises with correct alignment not only maximizes the benefits of each movement but also significantly reduces the risk of injury. For beginners, understanding and mastering form is essential before increasing intensity or volume in workouts.

Proper form ensures that the targeted muscles are being engaged correctly. For instance, in a push-up, maintaining a straight line from head to heels and keeping the elbows close to the body focuses the effort on the chest, shoulders, and triceps while protecting the lower back from strain. Conversely, poor form can lead to compensations where non-targeted muscles bear the load, which can lead to imbalances and potential injuries over time.

To achieve proper form, start by slowing down each movement. This allows you to focus on engaging the correct muscles and maintaining control throughout the exercise. It's also helpful to use mirrors or record your workouts to visually assess your form and make adjustments as needed. For those new to calisthenics, it might be beneficial to seek guidance from a trainer or use online resources that provide detailed breakdowns of exercise techniques.

Understanding Body Mechanics: Stability, Mobility, and Control

Calisthenics relies heavily on the understanding and application of body mechanics, which includes stability, mobility, and control. These three elements work together to ensure safe and effective movement during exercise.

Stability refers to the ability to maintain control of a joint or body position. In calisthenics, stability is crucial, particularly during complex movements like handstands or single-leg exercises, where the body must remain steady despite shifts in balance. Core stability is especially important, as it acts as the foundation for all movements, helping to protect the spine and improve overall performance.

Mobility is the range of motion available at a joint. Good mobility allows for more fluid and efficient movements, reducing the risk of strain or injury. In calisthenics, maintaining mobility in the shoulders, hips, and ankles is particularly important, as these joints are heavily involved in many exercises. Incorporating regular mobility exercises into your routine can enhance your performance and help prevent the stiffness that often accompanies repetitive movements.

Control in calisthenics is about the ability to execute movements with precision and smoothness. This is closely tied to the neuromuscular connection, where the brain communicates with the muscles to regulate movement. Developing control through slow, deliberate practice allows you to perform exercises with better form and reduces the likelihood of injuries caused by sudden or uncontrolled movements.

Warm-Up and Cool Down: Essential Routines to Prevent Injury

Warming up before calisthenics is non-negotiable. A proper warm-up prepares the body for the physical demands of exercise by increasing blood flow, raising body temperature, and improving joint mobility. This process gradually prepares the muscles, tendons, and ligaments for the upcoming workout, reducing the risk of injuries like strains or sprains.

A typical warm-up should last between 5 to 10 minutes and include both general and specific movements. Start with light cardio, such as jogging in place or jumping jacks, to get the blood flowing. Follow this with dynamic stretches that mimic the movements you'll be performing in your workout. For example, leg swings, arm circles, and bodyweight squats are excellent warm-up exercises that activate key muscle groups.

Cooling down is equally important as it helps the body transition from exercise back to a resting state. It aids in the gradual reduction of heart rate and helps prevent muscle stiffness by promoting the removal of lactic acid buildup. A cool-down should include light cardio, such as walking or slow cycling, followed by static stretching, where you hold stretches for 20-30 seconds to improve flexibility and relax the muscles.

Foundational Exercises

Mastering the Basics: Push-ups, Squats, and Planks

In calisthenics, foundational exercises like push-ups, squats, and planks are essential building blocks that form the basis of more advanced movements. Mastering these exercises not only helps in developing strength but also in understanding the fundamental mechanics of bodyweight training.

Push-ups are a comprehensive upper body exercise that targets the chest, shoulders, triceps, and core. Begin by placing your hands shoulder-width apart on the floor, with your body forming a straight line from head to heels. Lower your body by bending your elbows, keeping them close to your sides, until your chest nearly touches the ground, and then push back up to the starting position. Focus on keeping your core engaged and your body in a straight line throughout the movement. Variations like knee push-ups or incline push-ups can be used to build strength before progressing to the standard push-up.

Squats are fundamental for lower body strength, engaging the quadriceps, hamstrings, glutes, and core. Stand with your feet shoulder-width apart, and initiate the movement by bending your knees and hips, lowering your body as if sitting back into a chair. Keep your chest up, back straight, and knees tracking over your toes. Lower yourself until your thighs are parallel to the ground, then push through your heels to return to the standing position. Variations like wall squats or using a chair for support can help beginners perfect their form before progressing to deeper or weighted squats.

Planks are a powerful exercise for building core stability and strength. Start in a forearm plank position, with your elbows directly under your shoulders and your body forming a straight line from head to heels. Engage your core, glutes, and legs, and hold this position for as long as possible while maintaining proper form. Avoid letting your hips sag or rise too high. Plank variations, such as side planks or dynamic planks (adding leg lifts or arm reaches), can increase the challenge and engage different muscle groups.

Modifications and Progressions for Different Fitness Levels

One of the strengths of calisthenics is its scalability. Exercises can be modified to suit different fitness levels, making it accessible to beginners and challenging for advanced practitioners. Understanding how to modify and progress exercises is key to maintaining steady improvement while avoiding injury.

For beginners, modifications are crucial. If a standard push-up is too difficult, starting with knee push-ups or incline push-ups against a wall or bench reduces the intensity while allowing for the development of necessary strength and technique. Similarly, squats can be modified by using a chair for support or performing partial squats until full depth is achievable.

As strength and confidence grow, progressions can be introduced to increase the difficulty of exercises. For push-ups, this might mean progressing from knee push-ups to standard push-ups, and eventually to decline push-ups or plyometric push-ups for added challenge. Squat progressions could involve adding a jump at the top (jump squats) or holding weights for added resistance. In planks, extending the duration of the hold or incorporating dynamic movements, like shoulder taps, can significantly increase the difficulty.

Creating a Balanced Routine: Targeting Major Muscle Groups

Creating a balanced calisthenics routine is essential for overall muscle development and injury prevention. A well-rounded program should target all major muscle groups—upper body, lower body, and core—while incorporating elements of flexibility, mobility, and cardiovascular fitness.

A balanced routine might include the following:

Upper Body: Push-ups, pull-ups (or assisted pull-ups), dips, and inverted rows to target the chest, back, shoulders, and arms.

Lower Body: Squats, lunges, glute bridges, and calf raises to work the quadriceps, hamstrings, glutes, and calves.

Core: Planks, leg raises, Russian twists, and mountain climbers to build core strength and stability.

Additionally, it's important to alternate between different muscle groups in your workouts to allow for adequate recovery and avoid overtraining. For example, you might focus on upper body exercises one day, lower body the next, and then core the following day. Integrating rest days and active recovery sessions, like yoga or light stretching, helps prevent burnout and supports long-term progress.

By adhering to these foundational principles and exercises, beginners can build a strong base in calisthenics that will support their growth into more advanced movements and routines. This approach not only promotes physical strength and endurance but also fosters a deep understanding of the body's capabilities and limits.

CHAPTER TWO

Developing Strength and Endurance

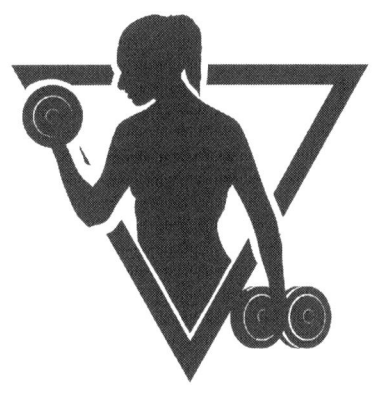

Strength Training for Women

Building Upper Body Strength: Pull-ups, Dips, and More

Building upper body strength is often a key focus in calisthenics, especially for women who may feel less confident in this area. Exercises like pull-ups, dips, and their variations are central to developing a powerful and functional upper body.

Pull-ups are a fundamental exercise in calisthenics, targeting the back, shoulders, and arms. They are highly effective but can be challenging, especially for beginners. Start with assisted variations, such as band-assisted pull-ups or using a pull-up machine, to build the necessary strength. Alternatively, practicing negative pull-ups, where you jump to the top position and slowly lower yourself down, can help you build the eccentric strength needed to perform a full pull-up. As you progress, you can move to unassisted pull-ups and eventually explore more advanced variations like wide-grip pull-ups or chin-ups, which place a different emphasis on muscle groups.

Dips are another crucial upper body exercise, primarily targeting the triceps, shoulders, and chest. For beginners, bench dips are a good starting point, where you use a sturdy surface like a bench or chair to support your body weight. As strength improves, you can progress to parallel bar dips, where you lift your entire body weight using dip bars or parallel bars. The key to dips is to maintain proper form, keeping your elbows close to your body and avoiding excessive forward lean, which can strain the shoulders.

Other complementary exercises include push-ups, which further develop the chest, shoulders, and triceps, and inverted rows, which are excellent for building the upper back and improving pull-up performance. These exercises can be scaled to match your fitness level and progressively made more challenging as your strength increases.

Lower Body Focus: Lunges, Glute Bridges, and Variations

Lower body strength is essential for functional fitness, supporting activities like walking, running, and lifting. In calisthenics, exercises like lunges, glute bridges, and their variations are effective for building strength in the quadriceps, hamstrings, glutes, and calves.

Lunges are versatile and can be performed in various planes of motion, making them excellent for developing lower body strength, balance, and coordination. Start with basic forward lunges, ensuring your knee stays in line with your toes and doesn't extend past them. As you gain confidence, progress to reverse lunges, lateral lunges, or walking lunges, which add dynamic movement and engage different muscle groups. Adding weights, such as dumbbells or a weighted vest, can further intensify the workout and promote muscle growth.

Glute bridges are a key exercise for strengthening the glutes, hamstrings, and lower back. Begin by lying on your back with your knees bent and feet flat on the floor. Lift your hips towards the ceiling, squeezing your glutes at the top, then slowly lower back down. This exercise not only builds strength but also helps improve hip mobility and core stability. Variations like single-leg glute bridges or adding resistance bands around your thighs can increase the challenge and target different aspects of the glutes and hamstrings.

Squats, while previously discussed as a foundational exercise, also play a crucial role in lower body strength training. Variations such as Bulgarian split squats (a form of lunge) or pistol squats (a single-leg squat) can significantly increase strength and balance, offering a progression path for those looking to further challenge their lower body.

Core Strengthening: Advanced Planks, Leg Raises, and Hollow Holds

A strong core is vital for overall stability, balance, and the execution of more advanced calisthenics movements. Advanced core exercises like planks, leg raises, and hollow holds target the abdominal muscles, lower back, and hip flexors, contributing to a well-rounded fitness foundation.

Advanced planks build upon the basic plank by adding elements that challenge stability and engage more muscle groups. Side planks focus on the obliques and can be made more difficult by adding hip dips or leg lifts. Plank variations such as plank-to-push-up or plank shoulder taps incorporate upper body movement, increasing the intensity and engaging the core in different ways.

Leg raises are highly effective for targeting the lower abs and hip flexors. Start with lying leg raises, where you lie flat on your back and lift your legs towards the ceiling, keeping them straight. To increase the difficulty, progress to hanging leg raises, where you hang from a pull-up bar and lift your legs or knees towards your chest. This variation not only strengthens the core but also engages the grip and upper body.

Hollow holds are a staple in gymnastics and calisthenics for building deep core strength. To perform a hollow hold, lie on your back with your arms extended overhead and legs straight out. Lift your arms, shoulders, and legs off the ground, creating a slight curve in your body while keeping your lower back pressed into the floor. Hold this position, engaging your core throughout. This exercise can be progressed by adding rocking motions or hollow body pulls to increase the intensity and challenge the stability of the core.

These core exercises not only build abdominal strength but also improve overall body control, making them essential for advancing in calisthenics.

Endurance and Cardiovascular Health

High-Intensity Interval Training (HIIT) Basics

High-Intensity Interval Training (HIIT) is an effective method for improving cardiovascular health and endurance, particularly when combined with calisthenics. HIIT involves alternating between short bursts of intense exercise and periods of rest or low-intensity activity. This approach maximizes calorie burn, enhances cardiovascular fitness, and can be completed in a shorter time compared to traditional steady-state cardio.

A basic HIIT workout might include exercises like sprint intervals, burpees, or jump squats, performed for 20 to 30 seconds at maximum effort, followed by 10 to 15 seconds of rest. A typical HIIT session lasts between 15 to 30 minutes, making it a time-efficient option for busy schedules. The intensity of HIIT triggers the afterburn effect (EPOC—Excess Post-Exercise Oxygen

Consumption), where the body continues to burn calories at an elevated rate even after the workout has ended.

For beginners, it's important to start with shorter intervals and longer rest periods, gradually increasing the intensity as fitness improves. HIIT can be tailored to individual fitness levels, making it accessible yet challenging for all.

Incorporating Plyometrics

Plyometrics, or jump training, is a powerful tool in calisthenics for developing explosive strength, speed, and endurance. Plyometric exercises involve rapid, explosive movements that generate force quickly, improving both muscular power and cardiovascular endurance.

Jump squats are a basic plyometric exercise that builds explosive power in the lower body. Start with a standard squat, then jump explosively as you reach the top of the movement, landing softly back into a squat position. This exercise not only strengthens the legs and glutes but also elevates the heart rate, making it an excellent addition to a cardio routine.

Burpees are a full-body exercise that combines strength, cardio, and plyometrics in one movement. To perform a burpee, start in a standing position, drop into a squat, kick your feet back into a plank, perform a push-up, then jump your feet back to your hands and explode into a jump. This sequence challenges the entire body and is highly effective for building endurance and burning calories.

Box jumps are another plyometric exercise that focuses on lower body power. Stand in front of a sturdy box or platform, bend your knees, and jump onto the box, landing softly with your knees slightly bent. Step or jump back down and repeat. Box jumps are great for building explosive leg strength and improving coordination and agility.

When incorporating plyometrics into your routine, it's essential to focus on proper form and landing mechanics to avoid injury. Start with lower-intensity exercises and gradually progress to more challenging movements as your strength and coordination improve.

Designing Circuits: Combining Strength and Cardio for Maximum Effect

Circuit training is an effective way to combine strength and cardio into a single workout, maximizing efficiency and results. In a circuit, you move quickly from one exercise to the next with minimal rest, targeting different muscle groups and keeping the heart rate elevated throughout.

A well-designed circuit should include a balance of upper body, lower body, core, and cardio exercises. For example:

Pull-ups (Upper Body)

Jump squats (Lower Body + Plyometrics)

Push-ups (Upper Body)

Burpees (Cardio + Full Body)

Plank with shoulder taps (Core + Stability)

Perform each exercise for 30 to 60 seconds, then rest for 15 to 30 seconds before moving to the next exercise. Complete 3 to 5 rounds of the circuit, depending on your fitness level and time available.

Circuits can be tailored to specific goals. For endurance and cardio focus, include more plyometric and high-intensity exercises. For strength, incorporate more bodyweight resistance movements with less emphasis on speed. The flexibility of circuit training makes it a versatile tool for improving overall fitness.

By integrating strength training, endurance work, and cardiovascular health into your calisthenics routine, you create a balanced and comprehensive fitness program that enhances all aspects of physical performance. This approach not only builds strength and muscle but also improves heart health, increases energy levels, and promotes long-term fitness and well-being.

CHAPTER THREE

Flexibility, Mobility, and Balance

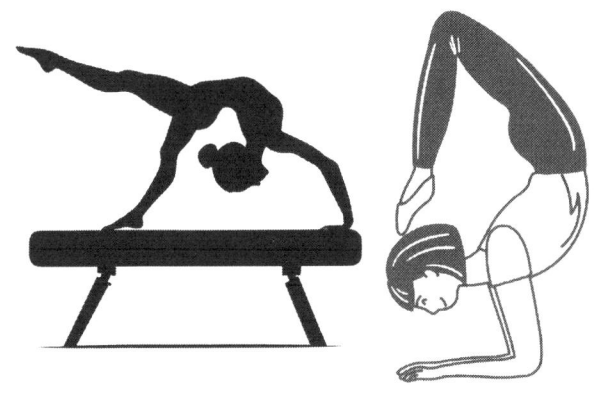

Flexibility and Mobility Training

Dynamic and Static Stretching: Techniques and Benefits
Flexibility and mobility are essential components of a
well-rounded calisthenics routine, as they enhance
performance, reduce the risk of injury, and improve
overall movement quality. Understanding the difference

between dynamic and static stretching is crucial for optimizing your training sessions.

Dynamic stretching involves moving parts of your body through a full range of motion, gradually increasing reach and speed. This type of stretching is ideal for warming up before a workout because it prepares your muscles and joints for the activity ahead. Dynamic stretches, such as leg swings, arm circles, and walking lunges, increase blood flow to the muscles, improve joint flexibility, and activate the nervous system. For instance, performing dynamic leg swings before a lower body workout helps loosen up the hip flexors and hamstrings, enhancing your ability to perform exercises like squats and lunges with better form and reduced risk of strain.

Static stretching, on the other hand, involves holding a stretch for an extended period, usually 15 to 60 seconds. This type of stretching is best suited for cooling down after a workout, as it helps to relax the muscles and improve long-term flexibility. By holding a stretch, such as a seated forward bend or a quad stretch, the muscle fibers are gently lengthened, which can improve flexibility over time and aid in recovery. Regular static stretching can also help alleviate muscle tightness, reduce soreness, and improve posture.

Both dynamic and static stretching play crucial roles in a comprehensive fitness routine. Incorporating dynamic stretches in your warm-up and static stretches in your cool-down ensures that your body is adequately prepared for exercise and supported in recovery, leading to better performance and fewer injuries.

Yoga-Inspired Movements for Flexibility and Recovery

Yoga and calisthenics complement each other beautifully, with yoga offering a range of movements that enhance flexibility, balance, and recovery. Incorporating yoga-inspired poses into your routine can significantly improve your overall mobility and mental well-being.

Sun Salutations are a great way to integrate dynamic stretching and movement into your routine. This sequence of poses, including forward folds, lunges, and upward-facing dog, stretches the entire body while also promoting blood circulation and improving focus. Performing a few rounds of Sun Salutations before or after a workout can help you transition between different exercise phases, keeping your muscles flexible and your mind centered.

Downward-Facing Dog is another yoga pose that stretches the hamstrings, calves, and shoulders while strengthening the arms and core. It's particularly useful in calisthenics for enhancing shoulder and hamstring flexibility, which is essential for exercises like push-ups and squats. Holding this pose for several breaths can help release tension in the upper body and lengthen the spine, contributing to better posture and reduced risk of injury.

Pigeon Pose is excellent for opening up the hips and stretching the glutes and hip flexors. Tight hips can limit mobility in exercises like squats and lunges, so incorporating Pigeon Pose into your routine can help increase hip flexibility and reduce discomfort during lower body workouts. This pose also promotes deep relaxation and can be particularly beneficial after a challenging workout, helping to ease muscle tension and improve recovery.

Yoga-inspired movements not only improve physical flexibility but also encourage a mindful approach to movement, enhancing the mind-body connection that is central to calisthenics.

Foam Rolling and Self-Myofascial Release Techniques

Foam rolling, a form of self-myofascial release (SMR), is an effective technique for improving flexibility, reducing muscle soreness, and enhancing recovery. By applying pressure to specific points on the body, foam rolling helps to release muscle knots, improve blood flow, and increase the range of motion.

To begin, select a foam roller with a firmness level that matches your comfort. Start with larger muscle groups, such as the quadriceps, hamstrings, and back. Place the foam roller under the targeted muscle, and slowly roll back and forth, pausing on any tender spots to apply sustained pressure. For example, rolling out the quadriceps can help alleviate tightness that might restrict movement during squats or lunges.

Foam rolling the IT band (the outer thigh) can also be beneficial, especially for runners or those who perform frequent leg exercises. This area can be particularly tight and may require gentle, prolonged rolling to release tension. By focusing on these areas, you can improve lower body mobility and reduce the risk of injury.

In addition to foam rollers, massage balls can be used for more targeted release, such as in the shoulders, glutes, or feet. These tools allow you to apply pressure to smaller, hard-to-reach areas that are prone to tension.

Regular use of foam rolling and SMR techniques can greatly enhance your flexibility and mobility, making it easier to perform calisthenics exercises with proper form. Moreover, these techniques help reduce post-exercise soreness, allowing for quicker recovery and more consistent training sessions.

Enhancing Balance and Coordination

Balance-Focused Exercises: Single-Leg Stands, Balance Board Workouts

Balance is a critical aspect of calisthenics that contributes to overall body control, stability, and coordination. Incorporating balance-focused exercises into your routine helps strengthen stabilizer muscles, improve posture, and enhance proprioception (the body's ability to sense its position in space).

Single-leg stands are a fundamental balance exercise that can be performed anywhere and require no equipment. Start by standing on one leg, keeping the supporting knee slightly bent and the other leg lifted. Hold this position for 30 to 60 seconds, focusing on engaging your core and maintaining a steady posture. As you progress, increase the difficulty by closing your eyes, adding arm movements, or standing on an unstable surface, like a cushion or balance pad. This exercise strengthens the muscles around the ankle, knee, and hip, improving overall balance and stability, which are essential for more advanced calisthenics movements like pistol squats or handstands.

Balance board workouts offer a dynamic way to challenge your balance and coordination. A balance board is a flat surface that sits atop a rolling cylinder or half-sphere, requiring constant adjustments to maintain stability. Exercises such as squats, lunges, or planks on a balance board not only target the primary muscles but also engage the stabilizers, enhancing joint stability and coordination. Regular use of a balance board can significantly improve your ability to control your body in unstable conditions, a skill that translates well into functional movements and sports.

Functional Movement Patterns: Improving Everyday Mobility

Functional movement patterns are exercises that mimic the natural movements of daily life, such as bending, twisting, reaching, and lifting. Incorporating these patterns into your calisthenics routine enhances your ability to move efficiently and safely in everyday activities.

Lateral lunges are an example of a functional movement that improves lateral mobility and strength. This exercise targets the inner and outer thighs while promoting hip flexibility and stability. By practicing lateral lunges, you not only build strength in the lower body but also improve your ability to move sideways, which is important for activities like stepping out of a car or moving quickly in sports.

Rotational exercises, such as Russian twists or standing wood chops, mimic the twisting motions used in many daily activities, like turning to grab something or swinging a bat. These exercises engage the core, especially the obliques, and improve rotational strength and flexibility. Including rotational movements in your routine helps to maintain a strong, stable core and reduces the risk of injury during twisting motions.

Hip hinge exercises, like good mornings or deadlifts, emphasize proper bending mechanics at the hips and are crucial for activities that involve lifting. These movements strengthen the posterior chain (hamstrings, glutes, and lower back), which supports proper posture and reduces the risk of back injuries. Practicing the hip hinge in a controlled environment prepares you for tasks like picking up heavy objects or lifting children, promoting safety and efficiency in daily life.

By integrating functional movement patterns into your calisthenics routine, you not only enhance your athletic performance but also improve your ability to perform everyday tasks with ease and confidence.

The Mind-Body Connection

Mindfulness, the practice of being fully present and aware of your body and surroundings, plays a vital role in calisthenics. Incorporating mindfulness into your training enhances the mind-body connection, improving focus, movement quality, and overall exercise enjoyment.

Mindful movement involves paying close attention to how your body feels during each exercise, focusing on the muscles being engaged, your breathing, and your form. This awareness helps you perform exercises with greater precision, reducing the risk of injury and maximizing the effectiveness of your workouts. For example, when performing a plank, mindfulness allows you to notice if your hips are sagging or if your core is fully engaged, leading to better alignment and muscle activation.

Breath control is another aspect of mindfulness that can enhance your calisthenics practice. Coordinating your breath with your movements helps regulate your energy and maintain a steady pace during exercises. For instance, inhaling as you lower into a squat and exhaling as you rise can help you maintain rhythm and focus, especially during high-intensity or complex movements.

Body scanning is a mindfulness technique that involves mentally scanning your body from head to toe, noticing areas of tension or discomfort. Practicing body scans before or after your workout can help you identify tight or sore areas that may need extra attention, such as stretching or foam rolling. This practice not only aids in recovery but also enhances your overall body awareness, making you more attuned to your physical state.

Incorporating mindfulness into your calisthenics routine encourages a holistic approach to fitness that nurtures both the body and mind. This connection fosters a deeper appreciation for the movements, increases exercise satisfaction, and promotes long-term adherence to your fitness journey.

By prioritizing flexibility, mobility, and balance alongside strength and endurance, you build a more resilient, adaptable, and functional body. This approach not only improves performance in calisthenics but also enhances your overall quality of life, allowing you to move with greater ease, confidence, and mindfulness in all areas of life.

CHAPTER FOUR

Crafting Your Personalized Calisthenics Plan

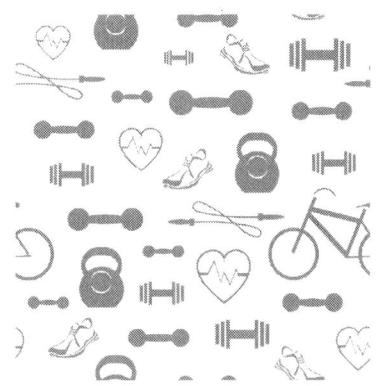

Assessing Your Fitness Level

Self-Assessments: Strength, Flexibility, and Endurance Tests

Before embarking on your calisthenics journey, it's essential to assess your current fitness level to create a personalized plan that meets your needs and goals.

Self-assessments in strength, flexibility, and endurance provide a baseline that helps you track progress over time and adjust your workouts accordingly.

For strength assessment, simple exercises like push-ups, squats, and planks can be used. For example, perform as many push-ups as you can with proper form to gauge your upper body strength. Similarly, see how many bodyweight squats you can complete in one minute to assess your lower body strength. Hold a plank for as long as possible to evaluate your core strength. Record your results to establish a baseline.

To assess flexibility, measure your range of motion in key areas such as the hamstrings, hips, shoulders, and spine. The sit-and-reach test is a common method for assessing hamstring and lower back flexibility. Sit on the floor with your legs straight out, and reach forward as far as you can. Measure the distance from your toes to your fingertips. For shoulder flexibility, try the shoulder reach test: reach one arm over your shoulder and the other behind your back, and see how close your hands come together. These tests help identify areas where you may need to focus more on stretching and mobility.

For endurance, a simple test like the 1-mile run or 3-minute step test can provide insight into your cardiovascular fitness. Time yourself as you run or walk a mile, and monitor your heart rate to evaluate how quickly you recover after exercise. Alternatively, use the step test by stepping up and down on a platform for three minutes, then measuring your heart rate recovery immediately afterward.

These assessments not only provide a starting point but also highlight your strengths and areas for improvement, allowing you to tailor your calisthenics plan to your unique fitness profile.

Setting Realistic and Achievable Fitness Goals

Setting goals is crucial for maintaining motivation and achieving success in your calisthenics journey. However, it's important that these goals are realistic, specific, and achievable to prevent frustration and burnout.

Start by identifying what you want to achieve with your calisthenics practice. Common goals include increasing strength, improving flexibility, enhancing endurance, losing weight, or achieving specific calisthenics skills like pull-ups or handstands. Once you have a clear idea of your objectives, break them down into smaller, measurable milestones. For example, if your goal is to perform a full pull-up, you might start with a goal to perform 5 band-assisted pull-ups within a month.

Goals should follow the SMART criteria—Specific, Measurable, Achievable, Relevant, and Time-bound. Instead of setting a vague goal like "get stronger," a SMART goal would be "increase the number of push-ups I can do from 5 to 15 in the next six weeks." This approach gives you a clear target and a timeline, making it easier to stay focused and motivated.

Remember to celebrate small victories along the way. Achieving these mini-goals reinforces your progress and keeps you motivated to continue pursuing larger goals.

Tracking Progress: Journals, Apps, and Other Tools

Tracking your progress is essential for staying motivated and adjusting your workout plan as needed. There are various tools you can use, from traditional journals to fitness apps, each offering different ways to monitor your achievements and stay on track.

Fitness journals provide a simple and effective way to record your workouts, including exercises performed, sets, reps, and how you felt during the session. Writing down your progress allows you to see improvements over time, identify patterns, and make adjustments as necessary. Journals also offer a space for reflection, helping you stay mentally engaged with your fitness journey.

Fitness apps like MyFitnessPal, Fitbod, or Jefit offer more advanced tracking features, including workout logging, progress photos, and even guided workouts. These apps can help you set reminders, track your nutrition, and connect with other users for support and motivation. Some apps also include progress charts and graphs, giving you a visual representation of your improvements.

Wearable fitness trackers like Fitbits or Apple Watches provide real-time data on your workouts, including heart rate, calories burned, and steps taken. These devices are particularly useful for tracking cardio and endurance progress and can be synced with fitness apps for a comprehensive overview of your activity levels.

No matter which method you choose, regular tracking helps you stay accountable, adjust your plan as needed, and recognize your progress, which is key to long-term success.

Designing a Beginner-Friendly Workout Plan

Structuring Your Weekly Routine: Balancing Strength, Cardio, and Rest

A well-structured weekly routine is essential for balancing strength training, cardiovascular health, and recovery. For beginners, it's important to start with a manageable schedule that allows for gradual progression while preventing burnout and injury.

A typical beginner-friendly routine might include:

3 days of strength training: Focus on different muscle groups each day (e.g., upper body, lower body, core), allowing each area to recover before being worked again. For example, you might train upper body on Monday, lower body on Wednesday, and core on Friday.

2 days of cardiovascular exercise: Incorporate activities like running, cycling, or swimming, or opt for a HIIT session that combines strength and cardio in one

workout. Cardio days can also include calisthenics-based circuits that keep your heart rate elevated while building endurance.

2 rest days or active recovery days: Rest days are crucial for recovery and preventing overtraining. Active recovery, such as light stretching, yoga, or a gentle walk, helps maintain mobility and circulation without placing stress on your muscles.

This schedule provides a balanced approach, ensuring that all aspects of fitness are addressed while giving your body time to rest and recover.

Sample Workouts for Different Goals: Fat Loss, Muscle Gain, and Toning

Your specific goals will determine the structure and focus of your workouts. Here are sample workouts tailored to common fitness goals:

Fat Loss: Combine strength and cardio in a circuit format to maximize calorie burn and maintain muscle mass. A sample workout might include:

3 rounds of:

15 push-ups

20 jump squats

30 seconds of mountain climbers

15 tricep dips

30 seconds of burpees

Rest 1-2 minutes between rounds.

Muscle Gain: Focus on progressive overload with higher resistance and lower repetitions. A sample workout might include:

3 sets of:

8-10 pull-ups (use a band if necessary)

10-12 push-ups (add weight if possible)

12-15 lunges per leg (holding dumbbells or weighted vest)

30-second plank hold

Rest 1-2 minutes between sets.

Toning: Emphasize endurance with higher repetitions and moderate resistance to create a lean, toned physique. A sample workout might include:

3 rounds of:

20 bodyweight squats

15 push-ups

20 glute bridges

15 reverse crunches

30 seconds of jumping jacks

Rest 30-60 seconds between rounds.

These sample workouts can be adjusted based on your fitness level and available equipment. The key is to stay consistent and gradually increase the difficulty as your strength and endurance improve.

Adjusting the Plan Over Time: Scaling Exercises and Adding Intensity

As you progress in your calisthenics journey, it's important to continually adjust your plan to keep challenging your body and avoid plateaus. Scaling exercises and adding intensity are effective ways to ensure ongoing improvement.

Scaling exercises involves modifying movements to either increase or decrease the difficulty. For example, once you've mastered standard push-ups, you can scale up to more challenging variations like diamond push-ups or decline push-ups. Conversely, if an exercise is too difficult, you can scale down by using an easier variation, such as performing push-ups on your knees or against a wall.

Adding intensity can be achieved by increasing the volume (more sets or reps), decreasing rest time between sets, or incorporating more complex movements. For instance, you might add a plyometric element to your squats by turning them into jump squats, or you could increase the duration of your plank holds to build greater core strength.

Periodically reassessing your fitness level will help you identify when it's time to scale up your exercises or adjust your routine to ensure continued progress. Aim to review and adjust your plan every 4-6 weeks, based on your goals and the progress you've made.

Staying Motivated and Consistent

Overcoming Common Challenges: Plateaus, Fatigue, and Time Constraints

Staying motivated and consistent can be challenging, especially when facing common obstacles like plateaus, fatigue, or time constraints. Developing strategies to overcome these challenges is essential for maintaining long-term success in your calisthenics journey.

Plateaus occur when your progress stalls despite continued effort. This can be frustrating, but it's a natural part of any fitness journey. To overcome plateaus, consider changing your workout routine by incorporating new exercises, increasing intensity, or altering your workout structure (e.g., switching from high reps/low weight to low reps/high weight). Periodization, where you cycle through different phases of training (e.g., strength, endurance, hypertrophy), can also help break through plateaus and reignite progress.

Fatigue is another common challenge, particularly if you're not allowing enough time for recovery. Ensure you're getting adequate rest, nutrition, and hydration to support your training. Listening to your body is key; if you're feeling excessively tired or sore, consider incorporating more active recovery days or reducing workout intensity until you regain energy.

Time constraints are a frequent barrier to consistency, but even short workouts can be effective if you're strategic. HIIT workouts, which can be completed in as little as 20 minutes, are an excellent way to fit in a high-intensity workout when time is limited.

Additionally, breaking up your workout into smaller sessions throughout the day (e.g., 10 minutes in the morning, 10 minutes at lunch, 10 minutes in the evening) can help you stay consistent without requiring a large time commitment.

Building a Support System: Workout Partners, Online Communities, and Mentors

A strong support system can significantly enhance your motivation and consistency. Engaging with others who share similar fitness goals can provide encouragement, accountability, and a sense of community.

Workout partners offer mutual support and motivation, making your workouts more enjoyable and less likely to be skipped. Whether you train with a friend, family member, or coworker, having someone to share your fitness journey with can make a big difference in staying committed.

Online communities are another excellent resource for support. Platforms like Reddit, Instagram, and dedicated fitness forums allow you to connect with others who are also on their calisthenics journey. Sharing your progress, challenges, and achievements with a supportive community can keep you motivated and provide valuable tips and encouragement from others who have been where you are.

Mentors or coaches can offer personalized guidance and feedback, helping you refine your technique, set realistic goals, and overcome obstacles. Whether you find a mentor in person or online, having someone with more experience to guide you can accelerate your progress and keep you on track.

Celebrating Milestones: Acknowledging Progress and Setting New Goals

Recognizing and celebrating your achievements, no matter how small, is crucial for maintaining motivation. Milestones could be anything from mastering a new exercise, reaching a specific strength goal, or completing a challenging workout routine consistently.

Celebrate your progress by treating yourself to something that supports your fitness journey, like new workout gear, a massage, or a healthy meal at your favorite restaurant. Acknowledging your hard work reinforces your commitment and reminds you of how far you've come.

Setting new goals after achieving a milestone keeps your fitness journey dynamic and exciting. As you progress, challenge yourself with new targets that push your abilities further, such as learning a new skill (e.g., handstand), increasing the intensity of your workouts, or improving your endurance. Setting new goals ensures that you continue to grow and evolve in your calisthenics practice, keeping your routine engaging and rewarding.

Crafting a personalized calisthenics plan tailored to your fitness level, goals, and lifestyle is a powerful way to take control of your health and well-being. By continuously assessing your progress, adapting your workouts, and staying motivated through challenges, you'll be well-equipped to achieve your fitness aspirations and maintain a lifelong commitment to physical fitness.

Printed in Dunstable, United Kingdom